BEFORE CALLING

THE DOCTOR

by

Phyllis Speight.

HEALTH SCIENCE PRESS
1 Church Path, Saffron Walden, Essex, England

By the same author
OVERCOMING RHEUMATISM & ARTHRITIS
ARNICA THE WONDER HERB
A COMPARISON OF THE CHRONIC MIASMS
A STUDY COURSE IN HOMOEOPATHY
HOMOEOPATHY FOR EMERGENCIES
HOMOEOPATHY, A GUIDE TO NATURAL MEDICINE
HOMOEOPATHIC REMEDIES FOR CHILDREN
PERTINENT QUESTIONS & ANSWERS ABOUT HOMOEOPATHY
HOMOEOPATHIC REMEDIES FOR WOMEN'S AILMENTS

ISBN 0 85032 137 9

Printed in Great Britain by
Whitstable Litho Printers Ltd., Whitstable, Kent

CONTENTS

FOREWORD

This little book has been written at the request of many patients during thirty years in a very busy practice. So many times I have heard 'We cannot find a simple book for beginners' and this is an attempt to help those enlightened folk who want to cope with the many ailments that do not need the attention of a doctor, at least at the beginning, but at the same time they do not wish to use the many pills and potions stocked by the orthodox chemists; in other words they wish to 'get away from drugs'.

Many serious illnesses have been aborted when the correct homoeopathic medicines have been administered at the onset of symptoms. I have seen many patients who had all the signs of developing serious troubles, but when the indicated homoeopathic remedies were given, they became well again, very quickly: and by this I mean not only were the symptoms removed but the feeling of well being returned and living was once again a joyous thing.

Homoeopathic remedies are safe, they do not suppress when used correctly, and they have no side effects.

I hope that many people will find this book helpful and, who knows, it may lead to more serious study in some instances.

Phyllis Speight.

THE PURPOSE OF THIS BOOK

'If he is no better tomorrow I must send for the doctor.'

It may be that little Johnny has a high temperature, or mother has influenza or perhaps father has a bad throat; it could be one of many troubles but the important question is what can be done during the next twelve hours to improve the condition in order that a visit from the doctor is not necessary?

I have tried to give clear indications for the use of some of the more common remedies that are so often employed in the treatment of everyday ailments.

We must forget our old habits of giving a name to the ailment and finding a bottle of medicine which carries the same name. Instead we must consider carefully the symptoms of the patient and match them as closely as possible to the most similar remedy.

No two people are alike and when sick they exhibit different symptoms. For instance if we look closely at three people suffering from influenza we find that the symptoms of one come on suddenly, the patient has a fever, is restless and fearful. The symptoms of the second took two or three days to develop, she is very tired and listless with chills running up and down the spine. The third patient has aching limbs, even her bones ache, and because of this she does not want to move; she too is shivering. The first patient needs aconite, the second gelsemium and the third eupertorium perf.

If you will read and study carefully the information given in these pages you will gradually become familiar with the remedies and then it will not be so difficult to choose the correct one when a member of your family becomes sick.

ABOUT HOMŒOPATHY

Homoeopathy is a system of medicine founded by Dr. Samuel Hahnemann over 200 years ago.

It is based on natural laws, one of which is that a substance will cure symptoms in a sick patient that it has produced in a healthy person.

A good example is that of a child who eats the berries of deadly nightshade (belladonna). He will exhibit all the symptoms of scarlet fever and belladonna (in homoeopathic potency) has cured many cases of this contageous disease.

All homoeopathic medicines are 'proved' on healthy men and women and there is no need for animals to be involved. Indeed our junior brethren cannot tell us how they feel and would be of little use in this field. Full details of this method are to be found in many homoeopathic text-books.

The preparation of homoeopathic medicines is a separate branch of pharmacy and therefore all remedies should be purchased from homoeopathic chemists. Details of potentization are also given in the many good text books.

Homoeopathic remedies may be obtained in the form of pills, tablets or tinctures but pills are undoubtedly the most popular. They will last indefinitely providing they are stored in a cool, dark drawer or cupboard away from strong smelling perfumes or soaps etc.

Owing to their sensitivity, potentised remedies should

never be transferred from one container to another unless the second one has already housed the same remedy in the same potency.

DOSAGE

I have indicated the required dose for the beginning of treatment in all cases but care must be taken to study the severity of the trouble and doses should be adjusted accordingly.

The golden rule is to stop the medicine as soon as improvement sets in and repeat only if the same symptoms return. If after a time there is no improvement in the patient then another remedy must be sought; this will show up more quickly in a very acute case such as diarrhoea or vomiting when improvement should be observed after three or four doses, whilst a good twenty four to thirty six hours may be necessary in indigestion or throat troubles and longer still in constipation and rheumatism.

If after a time fresh symptoms appear, then a different remedy must be found to match the new symptoms.

The pills should be taken into the mouth and placed under the tongue where they will dissolve very quickly and be absorbed into the blood stream.

TREATMENTS

ABSCESS

Belladonna 6 two pills hourly for a threatening abscess with redness, pain and throbbing.

Apis 6 two pills hourly when there is much swelling with stinging pain; there may be, in addition, redness, burning and throbbing.

Hepar sulph 6 two pills three hourly when matter has formed.

Silica 6 three hourly when suppuration has taken place but the poison is slow to come away.

Hot fomentations should be applied every two or three hours of a teaspoonful of calendula ϕ to half a pint of hot water. When the abscess has started to drain the fomentations should be reduced to two or three times daily.

(ϕ is the sign for a homoeopathic tincture.)

ACCIDENTS

Arnica 30 should always be given when any accident occurs, because not only does it deal with bruising of the soft parts, but it removes the shock and this is very important. But please note — arnica does not deal with shock from any other cause, see under 'Shock and Nervous Conditions'. The number of doses must be controlled by the severity of the case but two pills hourly for two or three doses and then less often according to symptoms is often sufficient.

Ruta 6 or 12 is the remedy for bruised bones and should follow arnica when required and given three or four times daily until improvement sets in.

Symphytum 30 should be given for broken bones after they have been re-set. This remedy helps the bones to knit together more quickly and lessens the pain. After an initial dose or two of arnica 2 pills of symphytum should be given daily (and I usually suggest bedtime) for two weeks.

Hypericum 12 or 30 should be used for nerve laceration or injuries to nerve endings such as finger tips, toes or coccyx (bottom of the spine). For the excruciating pain from shutting fingers in a car door a dose may be given at half hourly intervals for two or three doses and then less frequently. At the same time the affected part should be bathed with hypericum lotion made by adding half a pint of hot water to a teaspoonful of the ϕ. This remedy will prevent tetanus.

Ledum 6 or 12 should be used for 'puncture' wounds, such as splinters under the nail, or stepping on a tintack or when the garden fork is stuck into the foot. If given at once for a bad or dirty wound ledum will prevent tetanus. It should be thought of for any wounds that feel cold yet are relieved by cold.

Two pills may be given half hourly for three or four doses if wound is severe and then less often.

Ledum 200 is a routine remedy for a black eye and it will remove pain and discolouration quickly. It should be repeated only when necessary. A dose or two of arnica 30 should be given at the beginning of treatment to remove the shock of the accident.

Rhus-tox 6 or 12 is the first remedy to be thought of in sprains and should be given after arnica, hourly for two or three doses and then less frequently according to severity.

BACKACHE

Arnica 6 every three hours when aching is from over exertion such as spring-cleaning or playing tennis for the first time.

Aesculus hip 6 every six hours if backache with piles.

Kali carb 6 every six hours in pregnant women with a sense of weakness in the back.

Rhus-tox 6 or 12 every three hours for muscular stiffness from over-exertion or exposure to cold and wet.

BILIOUS OR STOMACH UPSETS

Iris versicolor 6 every two hours for nausea and vomiting of sour fluid that excoriates the throat. Sour vomit with headache. Vomiting of food an hour after eating.

Bryonia 6 or 12 every two hours when stomach is distended, with vomiting after eating. Patient must lie still, worse movement, nausea on sitting up.

Nux-vomica 6 or 12 every two hours for bad effects of coffee, alcoholic drinks, debauchery. Must loosen clothing. Vomiting of food. Stomach sensitive to pressure. Patient is irritable and often cold.

Natrum sulph 6 or 12 every two hours for constant rising of sour water. Nausea and vomiting with colic. Vomit sour followed by bitter liquids. Squeamishness in stomach before meals.

BOILS

Gunpowder 3X three tablets every three hours when there are no special indications.

Belladonna 6 every two hours when a boil is just beginning to form.

Silica 6 every six hours should be given when more advanced and pus is forming.

Arnica 6 every eight hours will act as a preventive when there is a tendency to boils.

BRUISES – See ACCIDENTS

BURNS

Urtica urens 30 and φ should be in every kitchen. When cooking it is so easy to burn one's hand or arm on the stove, or with steam from a saucepan or kettle. Very often applying the tincture at once is all that is necessary but if pain soon returns then a dose of the 30th potency will remove it. More tincture may be applied and the internal dose may be repeated as and when required. Of course any burns can be treated in this way but if very serious, then a doctor should be called in.

CATARRH

Bryonia 6 or 12 a dose every three hours for catarrh extending to front sinuses or into the chest. Offensive smell from mouth with hawking of offensive, tough mucus, sometimes in round, cheesy lumps the size of a pea.

Calcarea carb 6 or 12 a dose every four hours when nose is obstructed by yellow, fetid pus. Nostrils sore and ulcerated. At night nose dry and obstructed; by day it is moist and free. Catarrhal symptoms accompanied by great hunger.

Hepar sulph 6 or 12 every three hours – thick, yellow, offensive catarrh with inflamed swelling of nose which is painful, also pressure on larynx; hoarseness.

Kali bichromicum 6 or 12 every three hours. Catarrh with thick yellow or greenish ropy, stringy mucus (can be pulled out in long strings) or tough and jelly-like; offensive. Distress and fulness from inflammation in frontal sinuses.

Mercurius sol 6 or 12 every three hours. Catarrhal inflammation of frontal sinuses, nasal bones swollen. Greenish fetid mucus. This remedy should be taken by those with a general tendency to catarrh three times daily for two or three weeks, repeating at intervals.

Natrum muriaticum 6 or 12 every three hours. Mucus thick and like the white of an egg. There is much sneezing. Patients needing this remedy are often chilly and constipated and love salt.

Pulsatilla 6 or 12 every four hours. Green fetid nasal discharge with diminished taste. In chronic catarrh thick, yellow, bland mucus. Better in the open air. Nose stuffs up at night and indoors but fluent in open air. Loss of smell with catarrh. Patients needing this remedy are often tearful and they feel better in themselves when walking in the air.

CHICKEN POX

Aconite 6 every two hours in the early stages with restlessness, anxiety and high fever.

Antimonium tart 6 or 12 every two hours when vesicles form.

Rhus tox 6 every two hours if there is intense itching. Very often this is the only remedy required and when administered the symptoms soon disappear. When chicken pox breaks out in the home or at school, those not infected should take one dose of *rhus tox* 6 nightly for six nights.

CHILBLAINS

Pulsatilla 6 every six hours when there is a tendency to chilblains; patients with irritable skins; more painful when hot; in girls with painful or scanty menses.

Agaricus 6 three hourly when chilblains are more painful when cold.

Tamus φ applied locally with a brush night and morning is helpful.

Tamus ointment rubbed in night and morning at very first sign of a chilblain will often abort the trouble.

COLDS

Aconite 6 or 12 a dose hourly for three doses should be given at the sudden onset from exposure to cold or to cold dry winds. Fluent coryza of clear hot water and frequent sneezing. There may be headache, fever, thirst and sleeplessness. Doses should be given at longer intervals when symptoms improve.

Allium Cepa 6 or 12. This remedy is needed when there is streaming of the eyes and nose with headache; the profuse discharge from the nose is acrid corroding lips and nose; watering of the eyes, also profuse, is bland. Patient is hot and thirsty; worse indoors in warm room and in the evening. Better in the open air.

Arsenicum alb 6 or 12 every two hours. This remedy clears up a cold with thin watery discharge from nose which excoriates the upper lip, but the nose feels stuffed up all the time. Sneezing which does not relieve irritation in the nose. Head colds and sneezing from changes in the weather which often go down on the chest. Patient is chilly, likes to be near the fire, cannot get warm in spite of many clothes. He is restless, anxious and fastidious.

Bryonia 6 or 12 every two hours. Cold begins with a running nose, sneezing and watering, aching eyes and headache on first day; then it begins to travel downwards to throat and larynx with hoarseness; bronchitis may develop.

Camphor φ at the very onset when a person is thoroughly chilled and cannot get warm, two drops on a lump of sugar and repeated until warm will often abort a cold.

Dulcamara 6 or 12 every two hours is excellent for colds from cold, wet weather and snow; from getting wet or chilled when heated. Profuse discharge of water from nose and eyes, worse in open air, more fluent indoors in the warm, less fluent in cold air, or in a cold room. Sneezing worse in the cold. Eyes become red and sore.

Gelsemium 6 or 12 every two hours. Colds needing this remedy commence several days after exposure. Discharge makes nostrils sore and feel as if red-hot water is running down the nose. There are chills running up and down the back and the patient feels a great weight and tiredness of the whole body.

Nux Vomica 6 or 12 every two hours, for colds which come on in dry cold weather. Nose is stuffed up at night and in the open air; fluent coryza in warm room and by day. Sneezing. Patient is cold, cannot get enough clothes on and wants to hug the fire. Shivering from slightest movement or contact with the open air. This patient is usually very irritable.

COLIC

Chamomilla 6 every twenty minutes for pressive pain in stomach and under short ribs. Severe painful pressure in epigastrium making patient toss about in despair.

Colchicum 6 or 12 for colic worse eating and after flatulent food with great distention of stomach. Better bending double.

Colocynth 6 or 12 every twenty minutes for violent, cutting and tearing pains concentrating in the pit of the stomach, better from hard pressure and bending double.

Dioscorea 6 or 12 every twenty minutes for frequent sharp pains and burning, better belching. Sharp cramping pain in pit of stomach then belching of quantities of tasteless wind, better straightening up. Doses should be given at longer intervals as soon as there is an improvement in symptoms.

CONSTIPATION

Bryonia 6 three times daily when there is no desire; urging several times before results. Chronic constipation with headache. Stools hard, dark and dry as if burnt; large stools. Abdomen distended; rumbling yet obstinate constipation. The bryonia patient is worse for movement and irritable. He is thirsty.

Magnesia mur. 6 or 12 three times daily for constipation at the seaside. One of the key-notes of this remedy is worse salt, and the salt in the air by the sea causes constipation. Stools dry, they crumble at anus.

Natrum mur. 6 three times daily. There is obstinate retention of stools, irregular, hard and dry, often on alternate days. Does not know whether flatus or stool escapes. Constipation during periods. The natrum mur patient is irritable, weepy, hates fuss and craves salt.

Nux vomica 6 three times daily. There is urging for stool but it does not come. Sometimes a small stool is passed followed by a sensation that more is left behind; as if evacuation is incomplete. This remedy is often indicated for sedentary workers who are studious, extremely sensitive and very irritable.

Sepia 6 every four hours for ineffectual urging, stool not hard but much straining and sometimes sweating. Constipation of pregnancy. Feeling of a ball in the rectum which is not relieved by stool. Prolapse. The sepia patient is dull and indifferent with a tendency to prolapse, a feeling of heaviness and sagging.

Sulphur 6 every eight hours for stool only every two or three days which is hard, large and difficult. There is sometimes a sensation as if something is left behind in the rectum (like nux-vom) and there may be piles that bleed. The sulphur patient is warm, puts feet out of bed and throws off the clothes. He is hungry mid-morning.

COUGHS

Aconite 6 or 12 every three hours for constant short, dry cough with no expectoration; comes on suddenly after exposure to cold, dry winds. Wakens patient from sleep, dry, croupy and suffocating. Patient is anxious, fearful and restless. Worse at night.

Bryonia 6 or 12 every three hours for a hard dry cough with soreness in chest. Worse at night, after eating and drinking, and when entering a warm room. Cough compels patient to spring out of bed. Goes down to chest. Irritable patient.

Causticum 6 or 12 for hard cough which hurts whole chest. Inability to expectorate, patient feels if he could cough a little deeper he could bring up the mucus. Urine often escapes when coughing. Voice almost gone.

Pulsatilla 6 or 12 every three hours. Cough caused by inspiration. Worse warm room or coming into a warm room. Cough in the evening, worse lying down, prevents sleep. Paroxysmal cough from tickling in larynx. Dry cough, wants doors and windows open. Mucus thick bland, yellowish-green.

Rumex 6 or 12 every three hours for cough from breathing cool air; from changing to cold from warmth. Much tough mucus in larynx and constant desire to hawk without relief. Hoarseness. Dry spasmodic cough.

Spongia 6 or 12 every three hours. Croupy cough, sounds like a saw being driven through a board, with loss of voice. Chest dry. Wakens feeling suffocated with loud violent cough, anxiety and difficult breathing. Cough worse talking, reading, singing, swallowing and lying with head low.

CRAMP

Arnica 6 every two hours if cramp is in the calves from fatigue.

Cuprum 6 for contractions of muscles and tendons — a dose as is necessary and three times daily for a week following an attack.

Ledum 12 is excellent and often the only remedy necessary. Should be taken every ten minutes for three doses and three times daily for a week following an attack.

Nux vomica 6 every eight hours if cramp is from no special cause, coming on at night. May be repeated in the night if necessary.

A VISIT TO THE DENTIST

Gelsemium 30 a dose an hour before and a second dose just before going to the dentist calms the agitated person who gets worked up and sometimes develops diarrhoea.

Arnica 30 should be taken as soon after leaving the surgery as possible after extractions or fillings. Another dose or two may follow according to the severity of the treatment.

DIARRHOEA

Camphor φ two drops on sugar will often clear up acute diarrhoea if repeated every fifteen minutes.

Arsenicum alb 6 or 12 hourly for three doses and

less often as improvement begins for relentless purging often with vomiting; diarrhoea after eating ices or taking cold drinks when hot. Also after tainted meat, food or fruit.

Bryonia 6 or 12 every hour for three doses and less often as symptoms improve for diarrhoea in hot weather; vomits food; colic with thirst for long drinks; lumpy diarrhoea. Dry parched lips.

China 6 or 12 hourly for three doses and less often when symptoms improve for watery diarrhoea with much flatus; passes undigested food. Very debilitating.

Dulcamara 6 or 12 hourly for three doses and less often when symptoms improve for sudden attacks of diarrhoea in cold wet weather, every change of weather to cool. Colic as if diarrhoea would occur.

Podophyllum 6 or 12 hourly for three doses and less often as symptoms improve for profuse stools, offensive, gushing, painless. Desire for water but not for food.

DYSPEPSIA – See INDIGESTION

FEET ACHING

Arnica 30 hourly for two or three doses when aching from over-walking.

Arnica φ a teaspoonful in a bowl of water is very comforting when feet are bathed. This can be refreshing in hot weather.

HAEMORRHOIDS (Piles)

Aesculus hip 6 every four hours where there is much uneasiness, pain in back, constipation, general absence of bleeding but pain like sticks in rectum. Worse walking.

Causticum 6 or 12 every eight hours for hard piles, very painful when touched, walking, standing or sitting; better after a stool. Itching, stitching, stinging, burning and moist.

Hamamelis 3 every four hours for bleeding piles with loose stools. The rectum should be bathed with 30 drops of hamamelis φ in half a pint of water night and morning.

Nitric Acid 6 or 12 every four hours for piles which protrude and often bleed; burning and itching of anus; cutting pain after stool, constipation.

Nux-vomica 3 every eight hours for blind piles in persons of sedentary life, of costive habits.

Sulphur 6 eight hourly for bleeding piles, costiveness, feeling of faintness, sinking sensation mid-morning; worse at night on getting warm in bed and from washing.

HEADACHES

Two pills at hourly intervals may be given for the first three or four doses and then less often as improvement sets in.

Bryonia 6 or 12 for bursting or splitting headaches worse from any motion. Cannot sit up in bed. Worse any movement. Better lying still.

Gelsemium 6 or 12 for congestive headaches, pulsating. Neuralgic headache in temples and over the eyes, with nausea. Relieved by copious urination. Lies with head high. Feels exhausted.

Glonion 6 or 12 for waves of terrible bursting pulsating pain, worse bending head backwards. A good remedy for sunstroke. Worse for having hair cut. Worse heat about head. Throbbing head; head hot, face flushed.

Iris versicolor 6 or 12 for sick headache, has blur

before the eyes at commencement; nausea and vomiting. Vomit ropey.

Natrum muriaticum 6 or 12 for chronic headaches like little hammers in the head on slightest motion. Often begins at 10 or 11 a.m. and lasts until 3 p.m. or evening. Better for sleep. If very acute give Bryonia (it's acute) first and natrum muriaticum when the violent pain is over.

Nux-vomica 6 or 12 for headaches of sedentary persons; better when head is wrapped up. Feels as if a nail has been driven through brain. Stabbing pain with nausea and vomiting. Headache on waking; after eating.

Pulsatilla 6 or 12 for throbbing congestive headaches, head hot, better cold applications. Better slowly walking in fresh air. Periodic sick headaches. Headaches from over-eating. Headaches connected with menses or from suppressed menstruation.

HEARTBURN – See INDIGESTION

INDIGESTION

Carbo veg 6. Great distension of the abdomen with gas; belching with sour disordered stomach, constant eructations, flatulence, heartburn, waterbrash. Great accumulation of flatus in stomach, all food turns to wind. Relief from belching, constant belching.

Lycopodium 6. Pressure and discomfort in stomach after eating a *little* food. Must loosen clothing. Acidity, waterbrash, heartburn, fullness, flatulence, distension and bloating of stomach.

Typically this patient craves sweets and hot drinks, is worse from 4 - 8 p.m. Anticipates events such as speaking in public but is all right as soon as he begins.

Natrum carb 6. Greedy persons who love sweets and

nibbling. Much flatulence, always belching. Stomach sour. All gone feeling and pain in stomach which drives him to eat.

Nux vomica 6. After a meal flatulent distension. Nausea after eating, eructation of bitter and sour food. Flatulence rises and presses under short ribs. Putrid or bitter taste in mouth but food and drink tastes all right. Irritable patient.

Pulsatilla 6. From eating fat food; nausea with little vomiting; heartburn; feeling of distension, clothes have to be loosened. Patient is often weepy and is better in fresh air.

2 pills three times daily after meals in all cases.

INFLUENZA

Aconite 6 or 12. Sudden onset with fever; great restlessness from anxiety, sometimes with rapid heart beats and dry, painful cough. This medicine is needed when these symptoms come on after being out in very cold weather or cold winds.

Arsenicum alb 6 or 12 when patient has a bad headache, teasing cough which is worse at night, is restless with anguish and very fearful. Very often there is a high temperature.

Baptisia 6 or 12. Gastric flu, sudden attacks of diarrhoea and vomiting with great prostration. Face has a dark, patchy flush; patient is dull and confused and falls asleep while answering. Aching in all limbs; headache; restlessness.

Bryonia 6 or 12. The outstanding symptom of patients needing this remedy is that they do not want to move; they are worse from movement and want to be left alone and resent being disturbed. Thirst for long drinks of cold fluid at long intervals. Mouth and lips parched; dry hacking cough hurts the chest and head. Patient is irritable.

25

Gelsemium 6 or 12. The onset of flu calling for this remedy is gradual — perhaps two or three days. Patient looks drowsy with heavy eyelids, heavy head and heavy limbs. He is a tired patient. Chills run up and down back and during the fever there is no thirst. There is pain on moving the eyes and bursting headache from neck over head to eyes and forehead which is better by copious urination.

Eupatorium perf. 6 or 12. Intense aching in the bones of limbs and back, patient dare not move for pain. There is bursting headache, shivering, chills, vomiting of bile after drinking; great thirst, nausea, sneezing, soreness of eyeballs, watering eyes; hacking cough and hoarseness.

Remedies for influenza may be taken at hourly intervals for the first three or four doses and then at longer intervals as improvement sets in.

INSOMNIA

Arnica 30 a dose at bedtime from being physically overtired; body aches, cannot get comfortable, the bed feels hard.

Aconite 6 or 12, three doses at half hourly intervals at bedtime when there is anxiety, restlessness and patient is fearful. Sleeplessness of aged people; anxious dreams.

Arsenicum alb 6 or 12 three doses at hourly intervals at bedtime, for sleeplessness with anxiety and restlessness, tossing around the bed, cannot keep legs still.

Coffea 6 or 12 three doses at half hourly intervals at bedtime for sleeplessness from agitation, thoughts crowding into the mind, usually patient is worried.

There is every chance that one dose of the indicated remedy will prove successful so the mind should not be conditioned to the maximum number of doses. However if sleep proves difficult to capture, the indicated remedy should be taken three times daily for a week to ten days, the last dose being taken at bedtime.

LUMBAGO

Aconite 6 or 12 every two hours during the first day then less often as symptoms improve. Pain sharp as if beaten or sprained, from cold dry winds; from draughts. Lumbar region very sensitive.

Aesculus hip. 3 every two hours for severe, dull, aching pain making walking, stooping and rising from sitting almost impossible, often accompanied by constipation and piles.

Arnica 6 or 12 every two hours if from an injury. Back feels as if beaten.

Antimonium tart. 6 or 12 three times daily. Backache as from fatigue especially after eating and while sitting. Violent pain in sacro-lumbar region, the slightest effort to move causes retching and cold clammy sweat. Sensation of weight hanging on coccyx and dragging downwards.

Bryonia 6 or 12 every three hours. Pain worse from every movement, muscles painful to touch; bruised feeling in lower back when lying on it; worse from dry cold.

Rhus tox 6 or 12 every three hours for pains in small of back, better lying on something hard. Stiffness painful on motion; pain bruised or burning better during motion. Worse from damp, cold.

This remedy has the characteristic of stiffness and pains being worse on first movement but better after limbering up.

MEASLES

Aconite 6 every two hours when there is catarrh and high fever before the rash appears; subsequently itching, burning skin, rash rough, restless, anxious, tossing about, frightened.

Pulsatilla 12 every three hours when there is little fever, catarrhal symptoms, profuse lachrymation, dry mouth but seldom thirsty.

Euphrasia 6 or 12 every two hours when there is running from nose, streaming, burning tears, throbbing headache, dry cough and rash.

When measles breaks out in the home or school those not infected should take a dose of pulsatilla 12 nightly for six nights.

MENSTRUATION DIFFICULTIES

Aconite 6 or 12 three times daily for two or three weeks when period is late, diminished but too protracted. Plethoric females who live a sedentary life. Periods suppressed by fright with vexation.

Calcarea carb 6 or 12 three times daily for two to three weeks when period is too early; lasts too long and is too profuse induced by mental excitement or working too hard. Suppressed menses after working in water.

Natrum muriaticum 6 or 12 three times daily for two to three weeks. Menses too late and scanty, or too early and profuse. Before menses anxious, sad, qualmish; sweetish eructations in the morning; headache, eyes heavy, palpitation. During menses headache, sadness, colic. After menses headache.

Pulsatilla 6 or 12 three times daily for two or three weeks when menses is delayed and scanty, irregular, patient pale, languid and chilly. When periods do not appear at puberty and there is no local or constitutional disease to account for it.

Sabina 6 three times daily for two or three weeks. Menses too profuse, too early; flows in paroxysms; with colic and labour pains.

Sepia 6 or 12 three times daily for two or three weeks. Menses too early and too profuse; too late and too scanty; suppressed.

MUMPS

Jaborandi 6 or 12 every two hours. Should be given at the beginning of all cases of mumps as it so often clears up the symptoms, and removes the pain, before any complications set in.

Aconite 6 or 12 every two hours when there is fever, thirst and anxiety plus pain.

Carbo veg 6 or 12 every three hours if the patient catches cold during mumps and the mammary glands are affected in girls or the testicles in boys.

Mercurius cor 6 every two hours following aconite when fever has subsided.

Pulsatilla 6 or 12 every three hours if the testicles become affected and are swollen.

When mumps breaks out in the home or at school all those not infected should take Jaborandi 6 at bedtime for six nights.

NERVOUS CONDITIONS – See SHOCK AND NERVOUS CONDITIONS

OPERATIONS

Gelsemium 30. If worked up beforehand a dose at bedtime the previous night and another dose on waking on morning of operation. A third dose is permitted if necessary and if there is time.

Arnica 30 should be taken as soon after the operation as possible followed by three doses daily for three days.

PILES – See HAEMORRHOIDS

RHEUMATISM

Arnica 12 three times daily for two to three weeks for articular or muscular rheumatism, from exposure to dampness and cold; strained muscles due to over exertion. Limbs ache as if beaten; affected parts feel sore and bruised.

Bryonia 6 or 12 every four hours for heaviness of the limbs, they feel like lead (especially the lower), with redness and swelling of joints. Weakness of limbs compels patient to sit down. Worse on movement.

Colchicum 6 or 12 three times daily for two or three weeks for rheumatism in the small joints, tearing pains in muscles and joints.

Rhus tox 6 or 12 three times daily for two or three weeks for swelling and stiffness of joints from sprains. over-lifting or over-stretching. Pains in limbs with numbness and tingling; joints weak or stiff; shining swelling of joints. Worse on beginning to move and in wet, damp weather. Better from continued motion. Tearing pains in limbs during rest.

This subject has been dealt with fully in my little book *Overcoming Rheumatism and Arthritis.* (Health Science Press.)

SHOCK AND NERVOUS CONDITIONS

Arnica 30. Shock from accidents or physical injuries. Please note that this remedy will not deal with shock from any other cause.

Aconite 12. Shock from fear, it steadies the nervous system. (This remedy helped many people during the air-raids of the last war.)

Ignatia 30. Shock from grief or fright often with hysterical weeping and sometimes with fainting. It has helped many people after the death of a loved one.

Gelsemium 12. Nervous symptoms anticipating some event (like going to the dentist); examination funk; there is agitation, trembling and a feeling of limpness.

In all cases a dose should be taken at once, followed by one or two more at half-hourly or hourly intervals according to severity.

STINGS OF INSECTS

Ledum 6 every ten minutes and Ledum ϕ may be painted on the part, or ammonia applied.

STINGS OF BEES AND WASPS

Urtica Urens 30 every two hours.

Apis 30 every five minutes if there are symptoms of collapse in bee or wasp stings. If ammonia is not available the sting may be covered with a slice of onion which is very efficacious.

SLEEPLESSNESS – See INSOMNIA

STOMACH UPSETS – See BILIOUS AND STOMACH UPSETS

TEETHING BABIES

Chamomilla 6 is a wonderful remedy when baby is teething especially when one cheek is red and he is crying; does not know what he wants; as soon as you give him a toy he throws it down and wants something else. This remedy soothes and calms and has restored sleep to many parents in the middle of the night.

Dissolve three or four pills in a quarter of a tumbler of warm water and give a teaspoonful as a dose every twenty minutes until the baby is calm or asleep.

THROAT TROUBLES

Aconite 6 or 12. Throat very red, tingling. Acute inflammation which comes on suddenly (often in the night) after exposure to cold, raw wind.

Baryta carb 6 or 12. Every exposure to damp or cold brings on a sore throat with inflammation of tonsils, throat and fauces. It is slow to develop. Children with large tonsils who are intellectually retarded benefit from this remedy.

Belladonna 6. Inflammation of the throat; fauces and tonsils bright red and inflamed, especially right side, sometimes extending to left. Painful to swallow. Dryness of fauces. Aversion to liquids.

Patients needing this remedy nearly always have a congested, red, hot face and skin. Heat and dryness are marked.

Dulcamara 6 or 12. Sore throat from damp, cold weather; tendency to ulceration. Catarrh. Throat fills with mucus. Tonsils inflamed.

Kali bich 6 or 12. Tonsils swollen and inflamed; ulcers which tend to perforate. Discharges ropy, stringy and yellow which stick like glue.

Mercurius sol 6 or 12. Sore throat with every cold, smarting, raw. Discharge from nose yellowy green thick mucus. Tongue, thick, moist covering. Much sweating without relief. Worse at night.

Nux vomica 6 or 12. Sore throat; cold settled in nose, throat, chest and ears. Sneezing from itching in nose and throat. Sensitive to least draught. Patient is burning and hot but cannot move or uncover without feeling chilly. Often irritable.

Pulsatilla 6 or 12. Catarrh affecting throat which is bluish-red. Stinging pains worse swallowing saliva. Worse in warm air and room. Better cold, fresh, open air. Patient is sometimes weepy.

A dose of the appropriate remedy should be given every three hours until improvement sets in and then less often.

VARICOSE VEINS

Pulsatilla 3 every eight hours as a preventive or when an attack is feared. If there is much pain in veins this remedy should be given every two hours.

Hamamelis 3 every three hours when veins are enlarged and full.

Fluoric Acid 3 every four hours for long standing cases.

Hamamelis lotion should be applied night and morning. (30 drops of ϕ in half a pint of water.)

VOMITING

Bryonia 6 or 12 hourly. Vomiting of solid food immediately after eating. Nausea and vomiting in morning when waking; worse movement.

Ipecacuanha 6 or 12 hourly. Vomiting with *constant* nausea.

Nux vomica 6 or 12 hourly. Vomiting food and drink after overloading stomach. Usually feels cold and irritable.

Pulsatilla 6 or 12 hourly. Vomiting from a cold on the stomach or suppressed menses; after eating too much fat, pastry etc. Pale face with chilliness.

After three hourly doses longer intervals should be allowed as symptoms improve otherwise another remedy should be given.

The cause of vomiting must be ascertained and then treated accordingly.

WHOOPING COUGH

Arnica 6 or 12 is a wonderful remedy for a violent tickling cough which commences when a child gets angry. Begins to cry before cough; child knows it is coming and dreads it.

Bryonia 6 or 12. Child coughs immediately after eating and drinking then vomits; he returns to finish his meal and the same thing happens again. Dry, hard, spasmodic cough. Cough makes him spring out of bed.

Carbo veg. 6 or 12. An excellent remedy to be given at the beginning of whooping cough especially if child is fond of salt. Cough mostly hard and dry. Every violent spell brings up a lump of phlegm or is followed by retching and gagging, with very red face.

Drosera 6. Spasmodic cough with retching and vomiting. Often the only remedy required.

Kali carb 6 or 12. Convulsive and tickling cough at night. Cough violent and causes vomiting.

A dose of the indicated remedy should be given after every spasm of coughing.

When whooping cough breaks out in the home or at school, all those not infected should take drosera 6 night and morning for one week.

DIETARY HINTS

When suffering from colds, chills, influenza or any feverish condition it is wise to keep warm and have nothing but cleansing fresh fruit drinks for a day or two. This will help the body to clear out the toxins much more quickly than if meals are taken. As improvement sets in then light nourishing food may be added. This is especially important when nursing children and I have often been distressed to hear the mother trying to coax her child to eat. Nature usually dictates what is good for her and usually the sick child refuses food when feeling off colour. Fresh orange juice diluted with water, fresh lemon juice also diluted with a little honey added, or grapes when in season are excellent and all that is necessary until the temperature is normal and the patient feeling better.

It should be remembered that milk and dairy products are clogging foods and should be avoided in all catarrhal states.

To maintain health, all white flour and white sugar should be eliminated from the daily diet. Bread should be made from 100% wholemeal so that the wheatgerm, roughage and all the goodness is taken into the system. In some cases a change from white to 100% wholemeal bread is sufficient to cure constipation.

A little honey for sweetening when necessary (and barbados sugar when sugar must be used) should replace white sugar but cakes, biscuits and sweets should be cut to the very minimum. This is very important when bringing up children. I know many children who look upon an occasional sweet as a great treat; they are very happy to chew nuts and raisins or a carrot and their teeth are in much better shape in consequence.

Raw mixed salads should form part of the daily diet and extremely appetizing meals can be made by adding cheese, a few nuts or hard boiled eggs for protein. Plenty of conservatively cooked vegetables should be served with meat, fish or poultry, or a savoury if vegetarian. Potatoes should always be baked in their jackets to preserve the minerals which are just under the skin and usually removed with the peel. Fresh fruit should be taken daily.

Foods should be grilled, baked or steamed and not fried; and they should be cooked in stainless steel or ovenware and never in aluminium.

Far too many people take very little time in preparing food these days. Tins and packages are bought and heated in the minimum of time without any thought as to what these might contain (although the contents must be on the label!) or the balance of proteins, carbohydrates and starch.

If care is taken and *whole* foods prepared and cooked properly, much less sickness will manifest and a greater sense of well-being will be enjoyed.

SUGGESTED READING

PUDDEPHATT'S PRIMERS
by Noel Puddephatt revised by Phyllis Speight.
The three original Primers are now incorporated in one book which should be read by every beginner. Primer I — FIRST STEPS TO HOMOEOPATHY — introduces the subject and discusses how disease should be treated, what homoeopathy is; dose, potency and how to take the case. Primer II — HOW TO FIND THE CORRECT REMEDY — points the way to this difficult problem taking the novice through various stages of the valuation of symptoms, knowledge of the materia medica etc. Primer III is devoted to materia medica and includes the characteristics of thirteen leading remedies.
This revised edition is a 'must' for all beginners. Published by Health Science Press.

SIGN POSTS TO THE HOMOEOPATHIC REMEDIES
by Noel Puddephatt and Marjorie Kincaid-Smith.
In the Introduction Noel Puddephatt writes 'The dictionary tells us that a sign post is "a post supporting a sign; especially as a mark of direction at cross roads". It is at the cross roads where the student is most likely to go astray. The well proved remedies in the homoeopathic materia medica I have likened to cities and towns which may *look* superficially very similar to the novitiate; but to the experienced and the shrewd their essential dissimilarities are known and recognised'.
Seventy two homoeopathic remedies are written up in this way and it is an excellent book for the beginner. Published by Health Science Press.

HOMOEOPATHY FOR THE FIRST AIDER
by Dr. Dorothy Shepherd.
This is one of the most popular books on homoeopathy and excellent for beginners. Dr. Shepherd shows how to deal with many injuries and minor ailments and chapters include Treatment

of Wounds; Haemorrhages; Fainting; Burns and Scalds; Foreign Bodies in the Eye and in the Ear; Hernia; Poisons; Boils, Carbuncles and Septic conditions. The last chapter deals with potencies and dose and so the novice can learn a great deal from studying this book. Published by Health Science Press.

ESSENTIALS IN HOMOEOPATHIC PRESCRIBING
by Dr. H. Fergie Woods.

This book is a materia medica and a rapid repertory of the leading remedies. It enables domestic prescribers to select the correct medicine in a classical manner. A book for every beginner. Published by Health Science Press.

AN INTRODUCTION TO THE PRINCIPLES & PRACTICE OF HOMOEOPATHY 3rd Edition
by Drs C.E. Wheeler, M.D., B.S., B.Sc., & J.D. Kenyon B.M., Ch.B., L.R.C.P., B.Sc.

This book is intended for the student who wishes to make a serious study of homoeopathy. It supplies a technique for understanding the principles underlying the science. There are chapters on Materia Medica; The Principles of Homoeopathy; The Structure of the Homoeopathic Materia Medica; Homoeopathic Pharmacy, Potentization; Dosage; The Choice and Mode of Administration of the Remedy; Therapeutic Index and Repertory; General Index. Published by Health Science Press.

THE PRINCIPLES & ART OF CURE BY HOMOEOPATHY
by Dr. Herbert A. Roberts.

This book should be studied in great detail by every homoeopath as it presents a modern explanation of the basic principles of homoeopathy. This information is vital and should be known and understood by every prescriber. Chapters include Vital Force; Homoeopathy and the Fundamental Laws, Taking the Case; Analysis of the Case; The Law of Cure; The Dose; Remedy Reaction; The Second Prescription; Susceptibility; Suppression; Disease Classification. This is an official text book of The Hahnemann Medical College of Philadelphia. Published by Health Science Press.

HOMOEOPATHIC DRUG PICTURES
by Dr. Margaret Tyler M.D., L.R.C.P., L.R.C.S.

Dr. Tyler was a homoeopathic physician for many years working at The Royal London Homoeopathic Hospital as well as in private practice. She not only treated many hundreds of patients during her life but had a flair for teaching and this is why her 'Drug Pictures' is so popular.

Acknowledged to be one of the finest works for the study of materia medica, it deals with one hundred and twenty five leading homoeopathic remedies in an exciting way. She quotes other authorities in explaining their virtues and gives illustrative cases. Dr. Tyler gives a list of 'black letter' symptoms which are the important ones, culled from the great works of Hahnemann, Hering and Allen. Published by Health Science Press.

THE PRESCRIBER
by Dr. J.H. Clarke.

For over eight decades this book has been acclaimed as the most practical work of reference for the selection of homoeopathic remedies and this new edition is the finest yet published. The usefulness of this book is greatly enhanced by the inclusion of specific advice respecting potency and dose. All who buy this book should read the Introduction for sixty pages are devoted to lessons explaining the basis of homoeopathic prescribing which should be understood by all those using the remedies recommended. Published by Health Science Press.

SENSIBLE FOODS FOR ALL
by Edgar J. Saxon.

This book was first published in 1939 and has been in demand ever since. It covers a wide range of subjects appertaining to whole foods and should be of help to every family wishing to replace the present day packaged and processed food with a more natural, health giving diet. Published by The C. W. Daniel Co. Ltd.

TAKING THE ROUGH WITH THE SMOOTH
by Dr. Andrew Stanway.

Dr. Stanway argues in this lucid book that many of the great scourges of the Western world such as diverticular disease of the colon, constipation, appendicitis and haemorrhoids are preventable, and preventable in the simplest way, by certain changes in our eating habits, none of them difficult to achieve, none involving the painful self-discipline of going on a diet.

Many diseases are discussed. And it includes some delicious recipes. Published by Pan Books.

THERAPEUTIC INDEX

ACONITE

chicken pox; colds; coughs; influenza; insomnia; lumbago; measles; menstruation difficulties; mumps; nervous conditions; shock; throat troubles.

AESCULUS HIP

backache; haemorrhoids; lumbago.

AGARICUS

chilblains.

ALLIUM CEPA

colds.

ANTIMONIUM TART

lumbago; chicken pox.

APIS

abscess; bee stings; wasp stings.

ARNICA

accidents; backache; boils; cramp; dentist, a visit to the; feet-aching; insomnia; lumbago; nervous conditions; operations; rheumatism; shock; whooping-cough.

ARSENICUM ALB

colds; diarrhoea; influenza; insomnia.

BAPTISIA

influenza.

BARYTA CARB

throat troubles.

BELLADONNA

abscess; boils; throat troubles.

BRYONIA

bilious or stomach upsets; catarrh; colds; constipation; coughs; diarrhoea; headache; influenza; lumbago; rheumatism; vomiting; whooping-cough.

CALCAREA CARB

catarrh; menstrual difficulties.

CALENDULA

accidents; wounds.

CAMPHOR	colds; diarrhoea.
CARBO VEG	indigestion; mumps; whooping-cough.
CAUSTICUM	coughs; haemorrhoids.
CHAMOMILLA	colic; teething.
CHINA	diarrhoea.
COFFEA	insomnia.
COLCHICUM	colic; rheumatism.
COLOCYNTH	colic.
CUPRUM	cramp.
DIOSCOREA	colic.
DROSERA	whooping-cough.
DULCAMARA	colds; diarrhoea; throat troubles.
EUPERTORIUM PERF	influenza.
EUPHRASIA	measles.
FLUORICUM ACID	varicose veins.
GELSEMIUM	colds; dentist, a visit to the; headaches; influenza; nervous conditions; operations; shock.
GLONOINE	headaches.
GUNPOWDER	boils.
HAMAMELIS	haemorrhoids; varicose veins.
HEPAR SULPH	abscess; catarrh.
HYPERICUM	accidents; nerve injuries.
IGNATIA	hysteria; nervous conditions; shock.
IPECACUANHA	vomiting.
IRIS VERSICOLOR	bilious and stomach upsets; headaches.
JABORANDI	mumps.
KALI-CARB	backache; whooping-cough.

KALI-BICH	catarrh; throat troubles.
LEDUM	accidents; black-eye; cramps; insect stings; puncture wounds.
LYCOPODIUM	indigestion.
MAGNESIUM MUR	constipation.
MERCURIUS COR	mumps.
MERCURIUS SOL	catarrh; throat troubles.
NATRUM MURIATICUM	catarrh; constipation; headaches; menstruation difficulties.
NATRUM CARB	indigestion.
NATRUM SULPH	bilious and stomach upsets.
NITRIC ACID	haemorrhoids.
NUX VOMICA	bilious and stomach upsets; colds; constipation; cramp; haemorrhoids; headaches; indigestion; throat troubles; vomiting.
PODOPHYLLUM	diarrhoea.
PULSATILLA	catarrh; chilblains; coughs; headaches; indigestion; measles; menstruation difficulties; mumps; throat troubles; varicose veins; vomiting.
RHUS TOX	accidents; backache; chicken pox; lumbago; rheumatism; sprains.
RUMEX	coughs.
RUTA	accidents; bruised bones.
SABINA	menstruation difficulties.
SEPIA	constipation; menstruation difficulties.
SILICA	abscess; boils.
SPONGIA	coughs.
SULPHUR	constipation; haemorrhoids.

SYMPHYTUM	accidents; broken bones.
TAMUS	chilblains.
URTICA URENS	bee stings; burns.

TREATMENT INDEX